small change,
BIG RESULTS

The Trainer's Guide to Eliminating Childhood Obesity with Sports

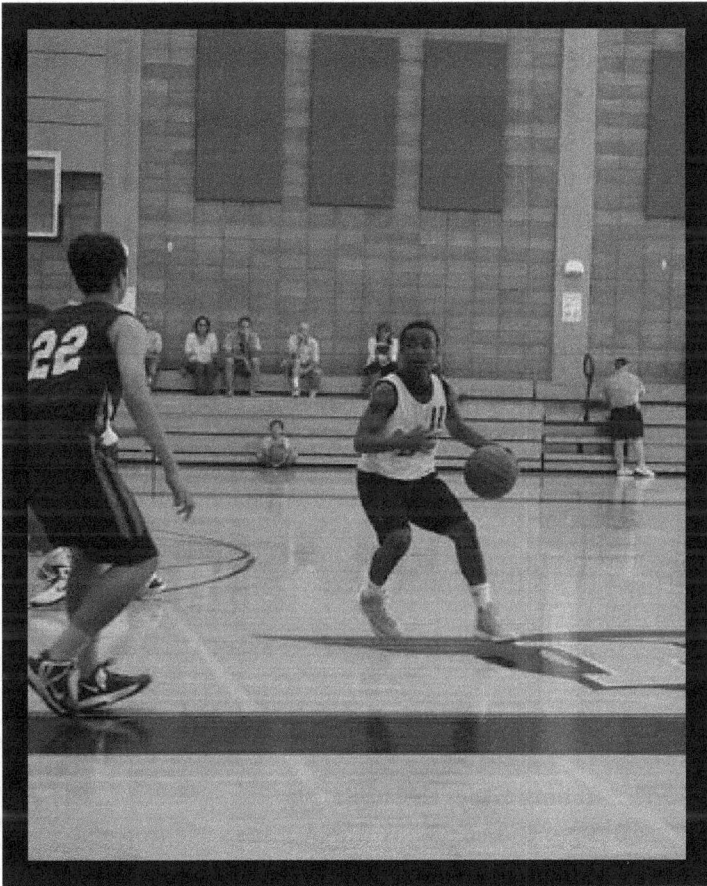

Cameron T. Russell
Myrtle D. Russell

small change, BIG RESULTS
Copyright 2013 Cameron T. Russell and Myrtle D. Russell
www.smallchangeguide.org

ISBN-13: 978-0615901657 (*small change* Press)
ISBN-10: 0615901654
Also available in eBook

Cover Photo: Cameron Russell
Cover Design: Elizabeth Little, Hyliian Design
Interior Book Design: Ellen C. Sallas, The Author's Mentor,
    www.theauthorsmentor.com

PUBLISHED IN THE UNITED STATES OF AMERICA

Preface

My dad was a mechanic, my brother is a mechanical engineer, and I work on bodies, so I guess I'm a body mechanic. Halfway around the globe and back, I have had the privilege of physically training individuals of all ages, sizes, shapes, occupations, and athletic backgrounds. From Super Bowl MVPs to pregnant moms, to weekend warriors with huge appetites for success, I have put them all through the paces in ways that suited their respective sports needs and fitness desires.

Through the years, the levels of fame, stardom and popularity that I have witnessed through my association with clients and patrons are stacked in my memory chest as high as the diminishing hair follicles on Shaq's head. I cherish the positive feedback moments picked up from the successes of my own "biggest loser" projects, just as much as watching a client such as Peyton Manning return from multiple neck surgeries to finish a season with a new squad he directed within two games of Super Bowl XLVII. I still recall vividly the many times that an overweight kid under my training instruction went back to win several medals in events at his school's "field day", although he had never been close to winning any event in previous years.

Those golden nuggets from Life have now spurred me to further my quest in changing the collective health of today's youth by encouraging parents to involve those possibly at risk kids in sports and physical activity. After all, as I continue to age, someone has to be around to help me with my groceries, listen to my stories, and make budding decisions for the future of this great country in which I choose to live.

The *small change: Big Results* project is an extension of the small change series my mother and I initiated in 2005. Within months of the initial release of *small change, a 28 Day Guide to Eating, Thinking, and Feeling Healthier*, I quickly grew tired of peeking into America's classrooms, having a hard time quickly recognizing the normally fit students. Less than twenty years ago, it was a much easier task picking out the overweight kid(s) in any middle school math class. Now the slim student sticks out like a Craig Sager suit on game night.

Seeking big results in the fight against childhood obesity, this venture ultimately spawned from the sheer desire to help others be healthy and live prosperous lives. After getting the balls rolling, doing interviews, and watching the words come together on my 32" Acer monitor (Huge right?), it quickly became an assignment to help parents and their children find healthy alternatives to the disturbing immobilization trend going on in way too many American households.

The age old adage, "An ounce of prevention is worth a pound of cure" isn't quite as stylish as it may have been when my grandparents still stood upright, but it still means the same thing for all in the 21st Century. Healthy, productive kids grow up to be healthy and productive adults, and normally those healthy and fruitful adults benefit from sustaining positive outlooks, living useful lives, and accumulating fewer healthcare expenses.

Take this tool and begin to make some small changes in your child's life by infusing sports and physical activity. Use it for the sole purpose of getting your child on the go and having fun. You will need time, a positive attitude, and a simple journal to note the positive, life-altering recommendations discussed throughout this book.

Be positive, have fun learning, and remain active!

Cameron T. Russell

Table of Contents

Introduction

Sports have been a societal mainstay for more centuries than we care to count. The Chinese engaged in sports as early as 4000 BC. Sporting activities became such a prominent part of Greek culture that the Olympic Games were created in the 8th century BC. From the first collegiate lacrosse game in the late 1800's, to the NFL's 2013 Super Bowl Sunday (the biggest annual sporting event held in the United States), Americans too have shared a great interest in sports.

With the emergence of mass media in the 1950's, sporting events were brought to America's living rooms. For the first time, families could enjoy unscripted athletic performances that would eventually create a national sports frenzy. The desire to emulate those performances opened doors for formal exercise in public schools, and in 1956, former President Dwight D. Eisenhower founded the President's Council on Youth Fitness.

But things were separate and not equal in public schools. Neither blacks nor females had equal access to the benefits of formal classroom physical education (PE). This would however change toward the later half of the 20th century with two landmark decisions in U.S. history; decisions that would usher in an even more rapid progression of physical education and sports throughout the country. The 1954 Brown vs. Board of Education Supreme Court ruling, along with the establishment of Title IX of the Education Amendment of 1972, made it possible for all students, regardless of color and sex, to participate in physical education. It eventually became a mandatory course in most middle and high school curricula.

But somewhere through the years Americans dropped the ball. The later part of the 20th century ushered in a decline in PE classes in many middle and high schools; a decline partly due to tighter budgets, a technological revolution, and increased focus on academics through such laws as the "No Child Left Behind" Act. Of equal importance is the fact that many PE classes became very formal and competitive. Students who were not the fastest and strongest were often ridiculed by peers and overlooked by teachers. Rather than advocate for policy changes, parents reacted by pulling their children out of PE classes, making it easier for the child to sit quietly on the sideline and avoid humiliation.

Unfortunately, students who continue to sit quietly on the sidelines or skip PE altogether have literally grown in size and number. The 2006 School Health Policies and Programs Study, a national survey conducted periodically to assess school health policies and programs, revealed that while 69.3 percent of elementary schools, 83.9 percent of middle schools, and 95.2 percent of high schools required physical education, only 3.8 percent of elementary schools, 7.9 percent of middle schools, and 2.1 percent of high schools provided daily physical education or its equivalent (150 minutes per week in elementary schools; 225 minutes per week in middle and high schools). Also worth mentioning is of the schools that required PE, 20.8 percent of elementary schools, 22.7 percent of middle schools, and 30.7 percent of high schools exempted students from PE requirements for high physical competency test scores; participation in community service activities; and participation in other school activities such as band or chorus.[1]

---

[1] www.naspeinfo.org

TACTIC ONE: Sports, Exercise, and Good Health - Making the Connection

"Sport is a preserver of health."
~Hippocrates, Greek physician; philosopher

While the nation's childhood obesity problem cannot be blamed solely on physical inactivity, it does carry some weight. As legislators push academics, school boards cut PE programs, and parents merely play "follow the leader," without question, the health of America's children is being "left behind." Lawmakers have dropped the ball by failing to realize the health benefits of physical activity, which can and should be fun and beneficial.

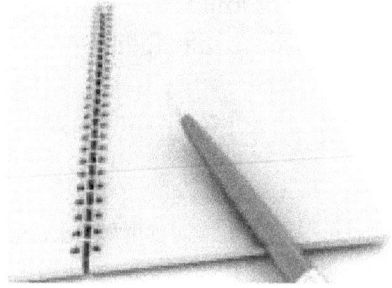

So we're stepping up to the plate to help you make sports and fitness fun for your children. In the words of the 39th president of the United States, Jimmy Carter, "Regular physical activity enhances both personal health and the vitality of our society. Establishing such an activity as a habit for all our citizens must be a national priority."[2]

Whether your child plays on a school or city-funded league sports team, or just likes to shoot hoops with neighborhood friends, sports offer so much more than just physical benefits. They help provide kids with academic, social, and mental building blocks that span a lifetime.

---

[2] Promoting Physical Activity: A guide for Community Action. US Department of Health and Human Services, Centers for Disease Control, 1999. Human Kinetics. pg. xvii

Children who participate in sports learn:

- Sports can be fun and prevent boredom.
- Leadership, socialization, and the value of relationships, as well as the value of teamwork.
- The importance of setting rules and how rules help maintain order in sporting events, as well as in life.
- To be competitive within a safe system.
- To develop self-esteem mastering skills that stressing the value of working to accomplish goals.
- Attitude control, self-discipline, resilience, and how to cope with adversity and disappointment.
- A feeling of belonging, balance, and a sense of community.
- Time management.
- The ability to think "long term." (Children who participate in sports learn the fundamental lesson of sacrificing immediate gratification for long-term gain, a basic skill for personal success).
- Life is give-and-take. (Sometimes you win and sometimes you lose, so be a good sport either way. Disappointment is no reason to give up).
- The value of diversity. Sports are a great equalizer: rich or poor, black, brown, or white, are irrelevant. (What counts is participation and heart).
- Respect for adults and peers.
- The impact that destructive behaviors such as drug and alcohol use can have upon their performance. (Therefore they are less likely to indulge).
- Sports are a good way to relieve stress and reduce depression.
- Motor skills, strategic thinking, and math skills.
- Regular exercise improves quality of life. (Children who exercise are more likely to continue the practice into adulthood).

Countless studies show that children who play sports, especially girls, are more likely to have a positive body image and higher self-esteem. They are also less likely to become overweight as adults, and the activity correlates well with a better mood, more overall energy, improved sleep habits and a stronger immune system. Plain and simple, sports exercise and good health mesh like peanut butter, jam, and two slices of whole wheat.

Cameron Russell:

At a time when overweight youth seem to litter the landscape of classrooms and communities across the country, a good old fashioned game of kickball could go a long way in preventing a growing number of tomorrow's "Biggest Losers." No, kickball isn't an official sport of the Olympics or X-Games, but it served as a great way for me and my grade school friends to stay active."

Myrtle Russell:

I started public school in 1959 in a rural West Tennessee town of about 9,000 residents. Back then, every student participated in physical education unless he was excused by a doctor. I don't remember seeing obese kids in my school. There were a few who were overweight, and usually they were the ones who dressed out for PE and stood around the gym wall complaining about why they couldn't do side straddle hops. They were also the ones who flunked PE and a few other subjects. By the time we reached high school, if they were still in school, they were overweight and still complaining.

small change A Activity to Kindle A Good Spirit:

Help your child develop an "attitude of gratitude" by starting a journal to promote being gratefully good and mentally healthy. Want to make it fun? Start one with him.

What does gratitude have to do with sports? Plenty. Athletes often base their self worth on performance, not understanding the difference between who they are and what they do. Getting your child to develop an "attitude of gratitude" early on helps him/her to see that there is much more to sports than winning. Enjoying the game should be the ultimate goal, minus the pressure to win.

Starting a gratitude journal is easy for both you and your child. Whether it's a Dora-theme pad with a lock and key, or a Detroit Red Wings spiral, treasure it!

After keeping a journal for a while, you'll be surprised at how many ways you and your child have been blessed, including within the sports and physical activity arenas.

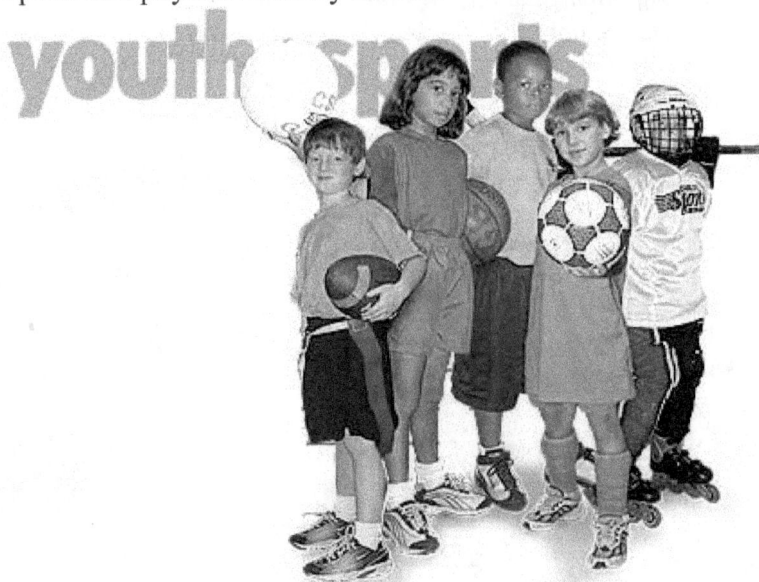

Here are a few more reasons for your child to adopt an "attitude of gratitude."

Gratitude:
- Fosters feelings of empathy and consideration for others.
- Is a life skill that can have a lifelong impact on overall happiness and well-being.
- Allows one to see how precious life really is.
- Reduces feelings of entitlement and chronic disappointment.
- Contributes to the development of resilience, which helps a youngster to withstand setbacks; rise to challenges; find new ways of solving problems; feel a sense of self-confidence; and know that hardship can be overcome.
- Teaches impulse control.
- Helps one to stay focused; usually the more focused one is, the better the performance.
- Teaches perseverance and patience; that certain things can only be obtained by working for them.

A grateful mind attracts to itself great things.

Cameron Russell:
I've spent most of my adult life gratitude journaling, but the thing I remember most about my first entry is how short and primitive it was. The only things I could think of to be thankful for were tangible objects that I could see, such as new sneakers, my truck, and a great roommate and best friend.

My list continued to grow each day that I consciously expressed gratitude, and I gradually began to understand that I needed to be more gracious toward the things and circumstances that I EXPECTED in my life. I began to pay the gratitude forward and watched my life change for the better as more and more of what I was thankful for started to appear.

At the time of my cousin's death, I wanted to scrap my last year of college and wallow in anguish, sorry, and self-pity. Gratitude journaling saved me from myself. I thanked God for graduating college each time I picked up my journal, and as expected...I did.

NOTES:

_____
_____
_____
_____
_____
_____
_____
_____
_____
_____
_____
_____
_____
_____
_____
_____
_____
_____
_____
_____
_____
_____
_____
_____
_____

TACTIC TWO: Promote Fun, Not Results

"In our lives we will encounter many challenges, and tomorrow we face one together. How we accept the challenge and attack the challenge head on is only about us--no one can touch that. If we win or lose this weekend, it will not make a difference in our lives. But why we play and how we play will make a difference in our lives forever." ~Beth Anders, 1984 Hockey bronze medalist and USA Women's coach

Before you read any further, ask yourself the following questions, which will help you focus on the benefits your child should gain from participating in sports. Think about each question for one minute, paying close attention to the answers that first come to mind.

Why do I want my child to participate in sports?

Will I be disappointed if he doesn't excel in a particular sport?

How will I react if he displays little or no interest in a sport I favor (one that I played or presently enjoy)?

Will I force him to continue even if it is no longer enjoyable?

There is no right or wrong answer, but no matter how you answered, your thoughts should have been centered around your child's benefits, not your own.

A single mom with a full-time career may simply want to

introduce her nine-year-old son to YMCA youth basketball to constructively occupy some of his "after school" down time. Her goal has nothing to do with making him the next Lebron James. Each week during winter's short days, the boy participates just for the experience of teamwork, occasionally mimicking some of Lebron's signature moves to the best of his ability. If his basketball talent matures to participation at the professional level, that is an added bonus. However, as long as the young dribbler takes pleasure in learning to shoot baskets, and refrains from negative behavior, - mission accomplished.

Regardless of your past experiences with sports, perhaps you were a professional coach or player, or you think pro wrestling is genuinely the best sport on the planet, as a parent, it's critical to remain focused on promoting sports as fun. No holds barred!

Restaurant Owner's Parental Plight

In 2008, Chattanooga restaurant proprietor Tony Ruiz realized it was time to consciously improve his family's health. Tony found himself spending far too many weeknights in the office of his bustling business, missing out on quality time family activities. With little physical activity, and constant exposure to high calorie foods, it wasn't long before Tony and his children began to pick up a few extra pounds. The weight gain led to general health and self-image issues, particularly for his pubescent daughter.

In a judicious father-daughter decision, with fun and fitness in mind, Tony signed his daughter up for soccer. He noticed a difference the opening minute of her team's first practice. The young female coach gave instructions and his daughter took off with the rest of the girls. He could immediately see that soccer would address her weight gain while improving conditioning; and serve as a shot in the arm to her self-esteem and body image.

Tony's daughter developed a liking for soccer that they both continue to share to this day. His initial idea had nothing to do with him loving soccer enough to pick up any and every goal broadcasting network on the planet. It had everything to do with his love for his daughter and concern for her well-being. She no longer plays the sport, but has no problem finding a way to get her soccer fix. She can always come in and help the crew down at the family's restaurant, and while there, find a game on one of the twelve plasma screens posted on the walls.

As parents, when you make the choice to add sports to your child's weekly activity wheel, be sure that you are doing it for the well-being of the child, and not for your own personal agenda. Remember, children mature at their respective paces, so steer clear of inflated expectations. Allow your child the opportunity to fully experience one of the last purist forms of enjoyment on the planet... Sports.

Cameron Russell

Your child's involvement in sports and any benefits experienced are just that...Your child's. So stay in the game by keeping your thoughts of grandeur out of the picture. As you continue to explore the activities in this book, keep your child's personal growth at the forefront of each decision you help them make. Whether your son scores a touchdown the first time he touches a football or your daughter scores her first goal in the other team's net, be open to allowing them to experience the rewards and consequences of participation.

Myrtle Russell

Both Cameron and my daughter Mia were athletes; both starters on their junior and senior high school basketball teams. They even tested their athletic skills in college, so I've attended my share of sporting events. I've seen parents get too emotionally involved in the game. You know, those who want to coach, referee, and play from the sidelines, firing insults at the coach and referee, often embarrassing the child to the point of wanting to quit the team. As a matter of fact, most children who quit sports leave because it is no longer fun; partly due to overzealous coaches, and parents who want to vicariously play the game through their kids rather than see things from the child's point of view.

When parents, who are obviously "out in left field," bring loaded guns to ballgames with intentions of bullying the coach into favoring their child, the wrong messages ring loud and clear: it's okay to blame others for your losses; there's nothing wrong with being a sore loser; bullying is acceptable; and I can take the law into my own hands without seriously thinking about the consequences of my behavior.

Instead the messages should be: enjoy the game; let the coach coach; it's okay to lose sometimes; it is a necessary part of life, particularly when you learn from your mistakes; and success comes with overcoming obstacles. It's just the way the ball bounces.

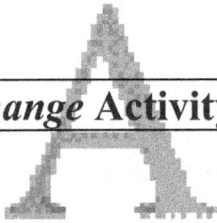

small change Activity to Kindle A Good Spirit:

Have your child write a "thank you" note to a person who has been especially nice to him in any setting. This could include a close friend, a teacher, or his favorite youth coach. "Thank you" notes benefit both the sender and the receiver. Don't forget to have him add it to his gratitude journal.

NOTES:

_____

_____

_____

_____

_____

_____

_____

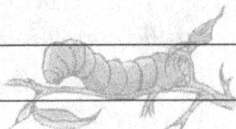

_____

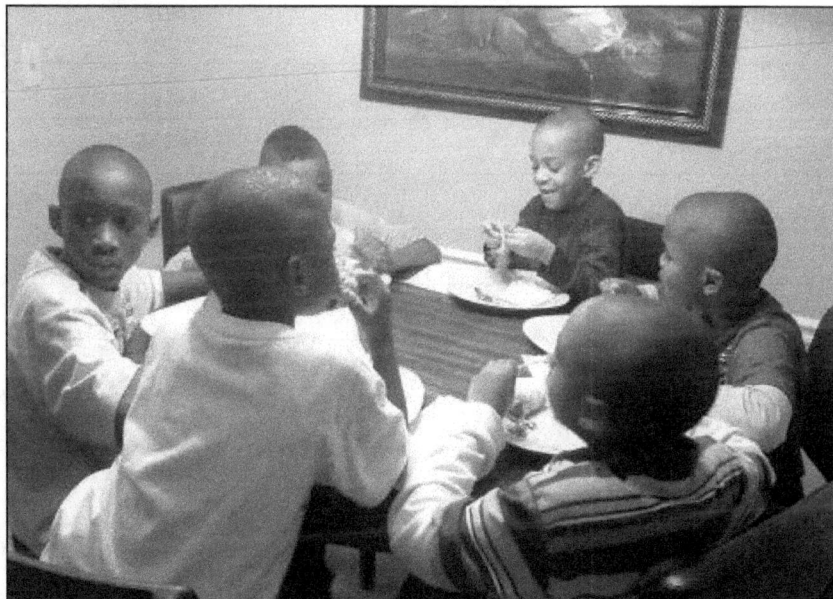

This crew of cousins enjoys a snack before a fun game of driveway holiday hoops.

TACTIC THREE: Sports Outlets- Plug in Anytime, Anywhere

"When I go out on the ice, I just think about my skating. I forget it is a competition." ~Katarina Witt, German Olympic figure skater.

Sports outlets exist by the thousands. Sparking your child's interest in a few of them takes less time than it does to nuke a bag of microwave popcorn.

The best way to influence participation in sports activities is to lay the foundation early by plugging your child into every available outlet you can get your hands on.

We offer four categories of sports outlets. By introducing children to any of these four categories, the parent becomes the positive influence in shaping a child's attitude about sports, rather than it being shaped by peers. You get the idea: act as if he/she already knows your highest expectations of her and it sort of becomes self-fulfilling. She/he becomes interested because you plant the seeds of interest in a positive, fun, and non-demanding way. For example: If your favorite NASCAR driver happens to be Danica Patrick, you could search out a copy of her *"got milk"* advertisement and show it to your daughter. At that moment not only is she thinking about her next glass of milk, she is also wondering why one of NASCAR's most popular drivers is sporting that funny milk mustache. Almost instantly you've helped her establish a connection to sports and possibly sparked her interest enough to want to learn more. It's that simple.

Remember: stay focused on the goal – fun and fitness. So grab a pen and note the four examples of ways to successfully plant harmless sports seeds into your child's consciousness.

1.   Sports Gear Presence

Anything used to play a sport of any kind is considered sports gear. Basketballs, hockey sticks, and cleats all fit the bill, but with the boom of extreme sports, even skateboards are now considered sports gear. (Be sure to wear proper safety gear.)

ESPN's Winter and Summer X Games winners get younger and more creative each year during seemingly heart-stopping competition. Twenty three year-old Shaun White has become extreme sports' main pitch by medaling in summer and winter X events.   White got his first professional sponsorship deal at age thirteen, and attributes his success to his mother's decision to put him on a snowboard during family ski trips at the age of ten.

From what I've been told, before I could officially walk, I was plugged into a small sports outlet. Perhaps my mom knew that putting a tennis ball in the crib would keep me busy and out of her hair for a while, or at least until it was time to stuff my face again. My mother had no idea that I would later serve MLB (Major League Baseball) and NFL (National League Football) clients as an adult, but she did recognize the immediate connection, which for me evolved from merely having a ball with a ball.

Later, those balls were joined by gloves, bats, skates, and other pieces of sports gear that helped make one of my first connections to sports enjoyable.

2.   Sporty Paraphernalia

From car keys to couches, almost any item can be emblazoned with a sports logo. Your child may associate his/her favorite logo with his/her favorite color, shape, or animal. Introduce a few if your child hasn't already adopted one or several, and see what happens.

Cameron Russell:
I personally chose a career involving athletics on many levels, and so almost seven days a week I'm dressed in sports gear such as warm-ups, ball caps, jerseys, or golf shirts. It all began as a toddler.

At the age of one, my mom had my first studio picture made at Sears & Roebuck. In that foggy looking picture that still hangs on her hallway wall, I'm outfitted in a velour track suit with balls patched on the front jacket pockets. The basketball, football and baseball on my jacket were nothing special along the lines of fashion, but seeing that picture daily always gave me a rock solid reason for gravitating toward sports influenced fashion. Every time my mother questioned my tastes while shopping, I reminded her of how she chose to outfit me in that picture. She caved every time.

3.   **Learn By Playing Sports Games**

Simulated sports are plentiful in the computerized gaming systems of the twenty first century. Companies such as X-Box, Sony, and Nintendo market a variety of sports-related games that are great teaching tools for introducing your child to sports. Beginners and novices alike are exposed to computerized activities that replicate the actual game such as Madden 2K10 (NFL football) or FIFA '10 (International futbol). The games' authenticity provides instructional tutorials and internet options that make playing the games easy.

Because playing simulated video games is a sedentary activity, be sure to monitor your child's sessions. You don't want to create an inactive video game junkie. Instead, your goal is to help your child understand the game of his or her interest.

Nintendo's Wii system offers even more gaming options for younger children. It provides them with a jump on hand-eye coordination and increased activity because of the semi-manual execution of movements required in each game. If the child chooses to bowl or swing a tennis racquet, he or she has to actually simulate the movement with the system's controller in hand. Now that dancing is also a sport, Nintendo Wii's *Just Dance* game is a great way to get your child moving in a healthy way, and offers a fun cardiovascular activity that you may enjoy as well.

Cameron Russell:

I met a seven year old boy who received his first Wii system as a Christmas gift. He instantly fell in love with tennis after playing it one time on a sixty-inch plasma television, and now takes lessons twice a week. He may never reach the skill level of ATP (Association of Tennis Professionals) superstars Andy Roddick or Roger Federer, but his interest peaked by believing that he was actually in the game as a great Wii tennis player. As a real participant in a tennis match, his confidence is as high as the empty hair follicles on Andre Agassi's head.

4.   **Sports Media Magic**

Newspapers, magazines, and broadcast media are awesome vehicles for sparking sports creativity and providing interesting information on athletes and their sports venue. Regardless of the age, exposing your child to sports related reading material, radio, and television broadcasts are solid foundations to build interest.

Reading to your children or having them read about sports in books, newspapers, or magazines, provides you with a great curiosity gauge.

Cameron Russell:

My inquisitiveness was sparked by having to read the sports page daily at the ripe old age of eight. Some lady that fed and clothed me suggested it as a way to make me a stronger reader. Not only did the extra reading develop my sports tastes, it also improved my reading comprehension and vocabulary. The more I read, the broader my sports loving horizons grew.

How's that for an added bonus or two?

Soon after developing some local journalism favorites, I got my first subscription to Sports Illustrated (SI). Although there was no Sports Illustrated for Kids in the eighties, I read original SI copies cover to cover, sometimes twice because they took me to places I never knew existed, sort of inspired creativity. That initial subscription led to twenty more, as well as the establishment of great reading habits.

In seventh grade, I even got a lesson in respect for authority just by looking at an SI edition during class time. Having completed my assignments for the day, reading extracurricular material during class time was no big deal for my teacher. As a matter of fact she encouraged it. However, on this particular day she was blown away by what I was reading. In my mitts I held a copy of Sports Illustrated's 1988 swimsuit edition, complete with spring sports and a few PG-13 photos of beautiful women twice my age.

"Put that away Cameron Russell. I can't believe you brought that kind of material to my class", said Mrs. Osler. "Where did you get that?"

Before she could get over to my desk I blurted a sinister response as if I'd been waiting on her to notice what she thought was racy content.

"My mother got it for me," I said with the conviction of a card shark holding a full house at Harrah's.

My classmates and I got the biggest kick out of an answer that left our beloved teacher standing with her mouth agape and no clue as to what to say or do. I did put the magazine away out of respect for her authority, and influence on my conduct grade, but the message at home did not change.

"Reading: It's fundamental."

There are countless ways to get plugged into sports, and we've only scratched the surface. Radio broadcasts and sports movies can also serve as substitutes to those we have mentioned in this chapter.

A *small change* Activity to Kindle A Good Spirit:

If your child is old enough to read, finding material is as simple as opening the sports section of your local newspaper. You can take it a step further by taking your child to your local library or bookstore to find reading material pertaining to sports and athletes. According to AllYouCanRead.com, *Sports Illustrated for Kids* ranks one of the top ten magazines for children in the world. They thoroughly enjoy the athlete interviews, comics, and splendid action photos that *SI for Kids* publishes.

If your child has not yet learned to read, introduce sports by reading to him or her an article on a particular athlete, or tune into a ballgame and watch the child's reactions. Better still, rent a few family-oriented sports movies and enjoy some valuable quality time, while establishing a connection to the wonderful world of sports. It's only a click away.

We've listed a few to get you started: *Rudy, Remember the Titans, Radio, Hoosiers, The Karate Kid, The Jackie Robinson Story, Bend It Like Beckham, Ali, Miracle, We Are Marshall, Pride, Rookie, The Blind Side. Coach Carter*

Put this fun activity in your gratitude journal at the end of the day.

Myrtle Russell: BACK FIELD IN MOTION

It was my younger brother Jerome that introduced Cameron to sports. I simply went along with the game. At the age of one, the first ball he ever held in his short, stubby little fingers had to be present. Well, he really couldn't hold it in his hand. He would hold it close to his chest, kind of like a quarterback cradles it in a game. By the time Cam turned two, his uncle began demonstrating stances and passing techniques. Most often his coaching would take place outside, but if the weather was bad and my mother was not home, he would turn her living room into a practice field, sometimes without her knowledge and always to her dissatisfaction. Jerome was passionate about passing on his sports finesse to his nephew and I think Cam just enjoyed the fun of it all. When he says that he literally grew up loving sports, it's true. He loved it so much that by the time he was four, against my strict commands to not leave the apartment complex, he would sneak off to watch the older guys in the neighborhood play ball, hoping, I guess, to be chosen to play on their team. But it would be three years and a few rounds of need discipline before that happened. At age eight, his wish was granted and he played organized ball for the first time with the North Yonkers Boys Club. For him I think it was sports heaven, his uncle Jerome was his proud personal coach and trainer.

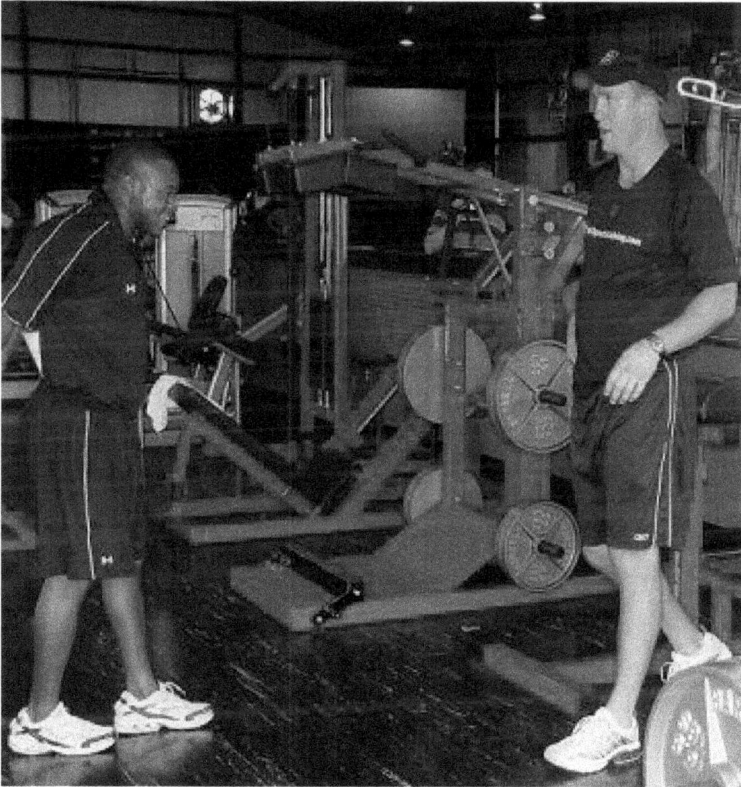

Peyton plugged into sports by first mimicking his dad. Maybe your son is running around the yard now imitating Peyton.

NOTES:

Time to Start Playing

"The values learned on the playing field--how to set goals, endure, take criticism and risks, become team players, use our beliefs, stay healthy and deal with stress--prepare us for life."
~Donna de Varona, 1960 Olympic Gold Medalist in Swimming

Regardless of the sport, picking the right place to start is crucial for your child's progress. Now that you understand the importance of sports and how to introduce them to your child, it's time to get a grasp on how to carefully choose the right level of competition for your child's personal sports development.

Cameron Russell:
When I first asked to play organized sports, the choice was a no-brainer. I would join the North Yonkers Boys Club because it was close to where I lived. It was the only organization in my neighborhood offering Pop Warner football and Little League baseball, and the opportunity for any boy on my side of town his first taste of teamwork, sanctioned competition, and the privilege of being togged up in uniform.

Today it's much easier finding an introductory league for your child than you think. With a click of the mouse you can research local leagues, find their locations, and subsequently increase your chances of finding qualified coaches and players having fun. Through your local newspaper you can also learn about league registration, whether its sponsored by a civic group, school, or a church.

• • •

Starting Blocks

As your child matures, several factors should be considered when choosing the right league to start a life long love for sports. Such factors include age, skill level, and in some cases size and weight.

On the introductory level, age requirements are usually first. A five year old gymnast is not expected to compete against a fourth grader on balance beams because her physical and mental maturity are years behind that of the older girl. She's yet to develop the necessary skills needed to successfully compete with the more experienced gymnast; therefore she should start with girls closer to her age.

There are body weight stipulations in many league by-laws, especially contact sports such as football, hockey and wrestling. These guidelines protect young athletes by insuring that they are not competing at a size or weight that creates a noticeable benefit or puts them at risk of being injured or injuring other players. Most contact sport leagues cover their bases by requiring that both the child's birth certificate and an updated physical be kept on file each season while participating.

Skill level is the final determining factor when placing your child in any organized sports league. Leagues sponsored by parks and recreation departments, community centers, and churches can be competitive and serve as great vehicles for learning the game. If your child openly displays more talent and skill than what is normally seen on the instructional level, seek out clubs or select teams that travel to face better competition. Organized soccer and gymnastic clubs are prime examples of sports that thrive on select teams and travel in efforts to increase exposure and improve play.

T-ball, a sport unbiased to gender, is the earliest level at which a child can be exposed to the basic concepts of baseball and softball. Because pitching of any kind is eliminated, the child participates without the fear of being hit by a pitched ball. Any child can begin playing at age four. By age eight the child generally moves on to a more competitive level of play such as Little League baseball or Pony League softball.

Lil' Kickers Soccer for Kids also provides a great opportunity for youngsters looking to cut their sports' teeth and participate without concerns for winning or losing. The same can be said for

The First Tee, a PGA youth development program dedicated to enhancing the lives of children through golf and character instruction.

Getting the Show on the Road

It's time to start using your resources. In addition to those previously mentioned, below are more examples of youth sports associations and programs focused on introducing children to sports and organized league competition. They're all easily found on the internet complete with league participation information, tips on getting your child started, and links to help you find a league nearby.

You can get the ball rolling by looking into organizations in closest relation to sports that interest your child. After you've gathered enough information, drop by the facility to look things over. Then talk with coaches and other participating parents about any concerns you may have related to competition, league by-laws and accountability. Also have your child interact with other players before making a sign-up decision. Remember, the goal is to find a league that fits.

Thanks to smart phones and the good people at *Google*, the statement "I don't know," is no longer an excuse for not taking action. Now pop any one of the following youth sports affiliates into your favorite search engine and get to work!

Upward Sports	*QuickStart Tennis*
YMCA Youth Sports	*USTA Jr. Team Tennis*
Jr. NBA/WNBA Basketball	*USA Gymnastics Clubs*
NFL FLAG Football	*Bassmaster CastingKids*
NFL Punt, Pass, & Kick	*USA Dance*
i9 Sports	*US Lacrosse*
TriFind Kids TriathlonsNat.	*Inline Hockey Association*
Youth Hockey Forum	*MLB's RBI Program*

small change Activity to Kindle A Good Spirit:

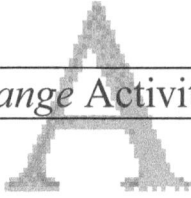

Have your child do a good deed for a neighbor, classmate, relative, or friend. It could be something as simple as taking out the trash, raking leaves, washing the car, or sharing a special game or toy with a classmate who is less fortunate. He or she could read a book to a young child, or try taking extra time to help a less skillful teammate get better.

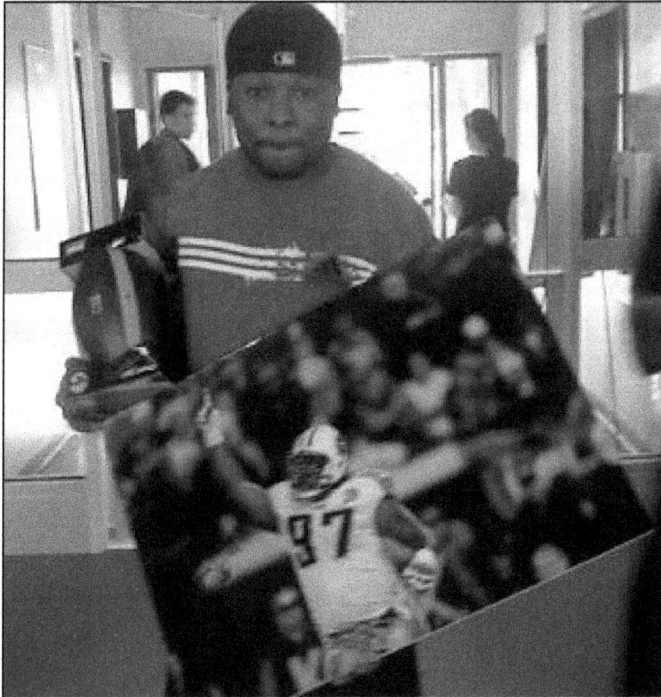

I've donated most of the memorabilia items I've collected over the years to charities that support many of the youth sports governing bodies listed previously.

TACTIC FIVE: Designate Rights and Privileges

Participation Comes With a Price

"Without self-discipline, success is impossible, period."
~Lou Holtz-retired coach; sportscaster

Now that you've researched your local youth sports governing bodies, it's very important that you enlighten your child to guidelines that he or she is to adhere to while participating in extracurricular activities. To have fun and be healthy should remain primary objectives for getting your child to love sports, but it is just as important for your child to understand that taking part in sports is a privilege. Whether your child is currently playing or not, this chapter from the *small change* creativity vault enlightens you to a few tried and true methods for maintaining the proper perspective.

So many athletes today view playing sports as being as much of a right of passage as taking their next breath. They've either never learned or forgot that playing any organized game for fun is a mere blessing. It is important that you get your child to understand this concept as soon as he or she has started participating in sports. Look at it this way- not only is your child going to improve his or her health and sports awareness by participating, he or she will begin to store up ounces of discipline that will accrue pounds of self-control and perspective as he or she matures.

One of my first recollections of learning responsibility occurred when I was nine years old and living in a Yonkers, New York housing project. As a Pop Warner football player at the North Yonkers Boys Club, I was beginning to make a name for myself as one of the better players in my neighborhood, especially the fall of my third grade year. After two games though, my season came to a screeching halt by way of my mother and her adamant approach to discipline in the home. At the time one of her favorite sayings happened to be "No instruction leads to destruction," and for her to have ended my season so abruptly was a clear indicator that I was not doing well with some of her instructions.

The black cloud began to appear as I consistently, but not purposefully forgot to do chores unswervingly enough for my mom's liking. Whether it was sweeping the floors, emptying the trash into the incinerator, or making my bed, delinquency seemed to rear its ugly head on every corner of my block. I found every excuse in the book as to why I so often forgot to take out the trash, or put my clothes in the hamper, but to my mom excuses were like hearts. (She used a slightly more colorful term.) Everyone has one.

On a brisk sunshiny fall day, I came home to our quaint box in the bricks and found all of my football equipment packed in a seemingly huge Hefty bag in the middle of the living room. As my mom stood in the kitchen preparing dinner after a double shift as a private duty nurse in Scarsdale, I asked the most pertinent question I could come up with at that moment.

"Why is my stuff packed up like this? We don't have practice for another hour," I said as I settled in at the kitchen table to do homework.

My mother's reply was quick and to the point, and she responded without even turning to look at me sitting there with eyes as big as the lights on the George Washington Bridge.

"Because you're having such a hard time handling your responsibilities around here, I'm relieving you of one," my mother said sardonically. "You are done with football until next season. Now take that stuff back to the Boys and Girls Club and tell Big Hutt why you can't play anymore".

Big Hutt, or Paul Hudson as he was known in the world, was my first and favorite coach of all time. He was a "player's coach" even in the mid eighties, but he wouldn't stand for his players disrespecting parents and mishandling responsibilities. Now that I had broken one of his commandments, I was totally embarrassed by having to quit the team due to selfish delinquency on my part.

The club was a ten-minute walk from our housing complex, but that day the walk seemed as if it took ten hours. The entire walk I cried and thought about what I could do to rectify the situation, but there was no use in all the contemplation. When my mom was out to teach a lesson, she did just that. I finally go to the doorsteps and quickly handed in my bag and scurried home before having to explain anything to the rest of my teammates who were already headed to the park across the street to practice. Big Hutt came by that night to ask my mom to exercise some leniency, but she flat out refused. He came by every week after that until the season was over, but to no avail. Myrtle Russell just wouldn't budge when it came to teaching life lessons and discipline.

My lack of responsibility cost me a year of sports and the neighborhood benefits that accompanied playing football, but I gained wisdom that is part of my personal intellect and make-up today. Without that lesson, I probably would have "forgotten" each day to responsibly write and share this nugget with you.

The Price You Pay

Regardless of the sport your child chooses to play, understanding that there are consequences for not following the standards for proper behavior and responsibility is vital. In addition to making sure chores are done and directions are followed in the home and at school, you can also set guidelines for healthy eating habits that encourage healthy living as they mature. Again, it's perfectly fine to enjoy treats like ice cream, fast food, and candy on occasion, but good health is as good health does. You can make sure that they are responsible eaters as adults by ensuring that they consume healthier foods as children. Be sure your child understands that participation in sports hinges on following directions and being responsible for his/her actions, both at home and away.

Cameron Russell

Remember the adage, 'No instruction leads to destruction' when your child starts to participate in recreational sports. Give him plenty of reign on the freedom rope, but the minute they break away from your set guidelines you have to quickly remind them that playing sports is a privilege and not a right. This includes ignoring home and school responsibilities and acting out at the wrong time and place.

A 'time-out' from participation, quiet time for reflection, and ultimately canceling the activity altogether are excellent ways to get the point across. Keep these ideas close, especially as your child matures and takes on even more personal responsibility.

Teaching youngsters about delayed gratification usually can be achieved by having them pick up toys or clothes and requiring them to study for longer periods of time as they age. Encouraging them to get jobs or save allowance money to pay for things they want promotes responsibility.

Myrtle Russell

Over the years, I've watched high school athletes excel to 'local super star' status. You know - the kid who gets the crowd roaring the second he walks onto the basketball court before he scores a basket, or the track star that gets the biggest servings of food in the lunch line, or the football jock that gets caught skipping class, but is spared punishment so he can play in the championship game. You get the picture?

For some athletes, both males and females, that same 'I'm entitled' behavior in school shows up at home and in other places. They come to expect special treatment. The son who skips class also skips chores at home and after a while, chores become a chore; he's much too important for such trivial stuff.

Super-stars don't have time to empty trash and make beds. After a while, in his immature egotistical mind, he is the boss at home just as on the court and before you know it, there is a loss of respect for parents and authority- a breeding ground for trouble. I've seen many athletes fall from grace and become stuck at the 'local super star' level, minus entitlement. Some are in jail and some on the streets where they tell their glory stories over and over until there's no one else to listen. Talented? Yes. Disciplined? No.

Remember the benefits of sports (Tactic One) and know that in many ways, playing sports is like participating in the game of life. Sometimes you win. Sometimes you lose. And everything you do comes with consequences and rewards. The earlier a child learns this, the better off he/she will be.

The mere fact that you can play sports is something to be grateful for. Think of all the people who would love to play but can't due to physical disabilities or economic hardships.

small change Activity to Kindle A Good Spirit:

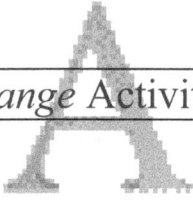

Start a year-long penny drive for a local homeless shelter, food bank, or your local youth sports association. Get family members involved. The more the merrier, and the more people you help (1,000,000 pennies = $10,000).

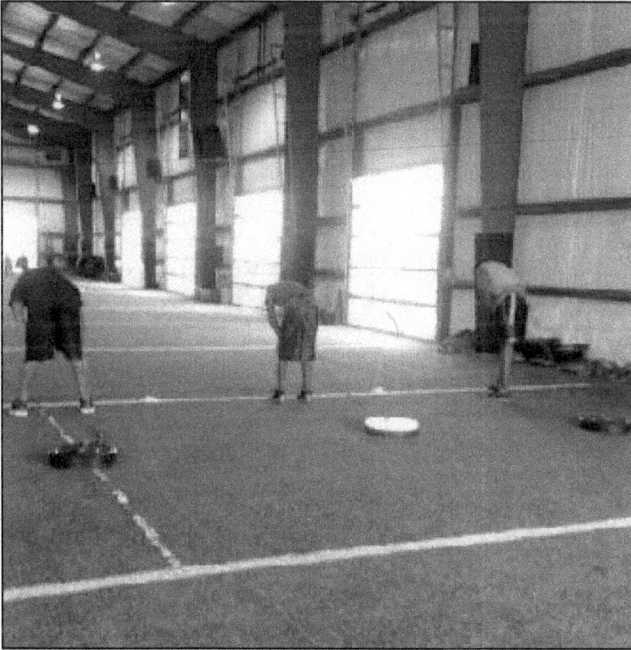

These Chattanooga-area prep athletes have been training with Cameron, and doing chores since age eleven. Now they are preparing for college, and only one is going to actually compete in sports.

NOTES:

Wins and Losses Are Minor for Children

"Victory isn't defined by wins or losses. It is defined by effort. If you can truthfully say, 'I did the best I could, I gave everything I had,' then you're a winner." ~Wolfgang Schadler-USA Luge instructor

No matter how hard it becomes to refrain from foreshadowing, try not to be consumed with outcomes. You have to be an advocate for giving 100% effort in practice and games, as well as reminding your child to exercise good sportsmanship. Remaining focused on exercise and having fun should always be the primary reason for your child participating in sports.

As a parent, winning and losing a game should be the least of your trepidations. Instead, encourage your child to enjoy the exercise and forget about who comes out on top.

Jay Cotton, Chattanooga advocate for the fight on childhood obesity, initiated a youth football program with intentions of targeting kids that normally would have a hard time cracking the line-up on many of Chattanooga's youth football teams. Ranging from age five to thirteen, youngsters registered as players on one of Cotton's Gateway to Opportunity (GTO) teams have greater chances of participating in an environment normally reserved for seemingly better athletes and more experienced players. Along with his NFL-veteran brother James, Jay and his staff make sure that each child involved in GTO's programs are well-coached and versed on the opportunities that await them on the field and in life. Cotton's kids may not be the best athletes initially, but they are treated as if they are. The Cotton brothers place special interest in fighting childhood obesity by schooling young athletes on healthy eating, getting exercise, as well as completing homework assignments and obeying their parents.

• • •

Whether he's conducting a youth skills camp in August or coaching a group of ten year olds in November, Cotton always manages to slip in promos for staying fit and being conscious of what's going into each of their young minds and bodies. Cotton doesn't get into the finer points of sports nutrition per say, but he definitely makes it a point to encourage more water consumption, less sugar intake, and increased activity.

Not one time have I heard either of the Cotton Brothers or their affiliates mention the words 'winning' or 'losing'. For people with a true desire to make a difference in the lives of young people, the only way to lose is to not try.

Promote Fun

Celia Kibler, co-founder and president of FunFit, Inc decided to get involved in the fight against childhood obesity after growing up as a youngster stuck in body braces in a battle with scoliosis (abnormal curvature of the spine). The 52-year old mother started Funfit as an adult fitness facility, but changed the company's focus to children without much of a background in sports and athletic activities. After redefining FunFit's services, Kibler realized that any child could have fun being active. It mattered little to Kibler that a child may have never thrown a ball or swung a bat before entering any of FunFit's fitness or sports-related training programs. With the heart of an elephant, and childhood memories of being left out of physical activities as a child, she was determined to squash one of America's biggest 21st Century challenges.

"Our programs are perfect for kids interested in or just starting to participate in team sports," said Kibler in May 2010, while on her way to an afternoon meeting. "FunFit's classes focus on continuous movement throughout the workout and go a long way toward improving coordination, overall conditioning, and even a child's cognitive skills. We've even seen test scores rise after consistent exercise and activity from many of our members."

Kibler, along with her Funfit staff, attack childhood obesity in a way that would make the Broncos' Peyton Manning blush. Kibler's creative methodology is right on target for eliminating one of America's biggest epidemics, but isn't necessarily in the business of producing future super Bowl MVPs. Try D1 Sports Training for that. However, Funfit does encourage kids to participate in sports and sports related activities. The Rockville, MD, based facility even services local sports teams looking for a training session focused on continuous movement.

"We (Funfit) are always encouraging coaches and teams to come in and work out on our circuit program. It offers the coach and his/her team a change of pace."

Learn more about Funfit's programs and locations at www.funfit.us, or plug "family fitness" into your favorite internet search engine and get information on facilities with a similar approach near you.

It's About the Journey, Not the Destination

My young cousin, Calvin Martin had the awesome experience of playing his first Pop Warner football game in the San Diego Chargers' spacious confines. The 21st Century "Beaver Cleaver" hadn't strapped on pads before the fall of 2010, but knowing his team was THE halftime show during a Charger preseason game was plenty of motivation to mix it up.

Before deciding to play that season at age 10, Calvin had no idea he'd be sharing turf with Charger QB Phillip Rivers. Now he's glad our sports enthused uncle slightly coerced him into signing up to play for the Rancho Bernardo Broncos. Not only did Calvin get to run around before 60,000 people, he got close enough to size up a guy not much taller than himself in then-Charger running back, Darren Sproles. The diminutive speed merchant gave Cal a high-five as he left the field.

Practicing three times a week and playing games on Saturday will take care of the exercise that Calvin needs, but the experience he gained from giving sports a chance will last a lifetime. When asked the following day how his team fared in Qualcomm Stadium via telephone, courageous Calvin had already forgotten the score. All he could talk about was going to his next practice.

In essence, wins and losses have absolutely nothing to do with how much fun a kid has playing an organized game in which exercise is the primary benefit. Positive memories and a boost to the self-image are added bonuses, but being involved for the shear enjoyment of the situation is so much more gratifying than who topped who on the scoreboard. In 36 years on this planet, I've never witnessed a Little League, Pop Warner, or YMCA coach get canned for losing.

small change Activity to Kindle A Good Spirit:

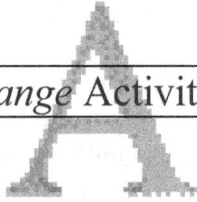

The next time your child prepares for game day, plant seeds of encouragement and enjoyment. Instead of statements such as "I hope you guys win today," or "Make sure you shoot the ball 20 times," try to reinforce having fun with the following statements.

"I'm going to have so much fun watching you play."

"Do what you do best today."

"You only lose when you fail to do the best you can."

"I love you, win or lose."

Asking some of the following questions post-game will imprint on your child's mind the importance of giving maximum effort in all areas and fostering creative thoughts.

"What did you like most about today's game/practice?"

"Did you have fun?"

"Are you tired after all the running around you did?"

"Wow, you guys really played as a team. Are you going to play that hard the next game too?

TACTIC SEVEN: Be a Fan

Let Coaches Coach, Players Play

"If you trust, you will be disappointed occasionally, but if you mistrust, you will be miserable all the time."
~Abraham Lincoln

One of the biggest challenges for youth sports coaches involves dealing with unruly parents overstepping their boundaries from the sidelines. Way too often some coach is trying to instruct a team or individual, and has to talk over or tune out the added directions of a parent that can't quite separate encouragement from interference. The usually unpaid coach is present to help youngsters feel good about themselves and live healthier lives, as well as provide instruction, but many parents often lose sight of that.

Supporting your child in efforts to get them fit and to promote fun is one thing, but trying to be Phil Jackson from the stands while your child's coach is teaching a fundamental lay-up is another. In order to keep your kid interested in sports and vigor under his or her own free will, you have to willingly allow coaches to coach and let players play.

The J.A. Henry YMCA in Chattanooga provided me with my first youth coaching experience nearly a decade ago, but several issues that surfaced then are still concerns now. I was asked to coach a co-ed basketball team of seven and eight year olds scheduled to compete in an all-boys league, but the challenge was magnetic, so I accepted. As a first time coach in my early twenties, I had no way of knowing how enthralled parents can become when watching their kids compete. After I took the post and scheduled

● ● ●

the first practice, roadblocks began to appear.

Obviously, the first concern happened to be the challenge of getting my players into better cardiovascular shape. Basketball requires movement in order to enjoy participation, so getting them used to running and jumping consistently was first priority. I had to stress to them the importance of exercise by explaining to them that being in great shape gives them energy to do more of what they like to do on the court.

Teaching basic dribbling, passing, and shooting drills was a patience-filled given; but the second biggest hurdle came by way of parents complaining about their child's playing time, or giving contradictory instruction from the stands. Not many parents stuck around to endure hour-long practices packed with fundamentals, but nearly all were present on Saturday mornings to witness the perceived progress. It's as if they were expecting Kobe Bryant or Candace Parker to show up reincarnated as their child on game-day.

Parker's Plight

One boy I'll refer to as "Parker" showed an uncanny ability to get shots off, not to mention exceptional athleticism for that age group, but he hadn't quite mastered the nuances of good ball-handling. Parker was as quick as a cat dodging raindrops, but was doing what eight year-olds do when picking up a basketball for the first time. He too ran with the ball instead of initially taking a dribble or three before shooting a lay-up.

Because Parker made twice the shots as his teammates, and stole almost every ball he could get his diminutive hands on, Parker's mom thought it was a good idea to move her son up a level with total disregard for his peer development and confidence. After three games, I noticed Parker practicing with the nine and ten year old team without the same smile he often displayed while running around with the kids he looked eyeball to eyeball. He was shorter than most of his new teammates and opponents and not as skilled or experienced for that level of competition. On that level, Parker was expected to travel less, dribble more, and exercise a higher basketball I.Q. Parker virtually lost a year of fun because his mother may have overstepped her sports knowledge boundaries.

It's easy to see why parents get a bit carried away with their children's involvement in sports, but again remembering the reason for the season is always pertinent. Exercise and having fun are the baselines for participation no matter what outside influences may creep into your peripheral. One of the best ways to trick your child into exercising is by slipping him into sports, but be sure not to ruin the experience with undue pressure.

Wesley's World of Support

Wesley, an 11-year-old basketball buff in Memphis, started shooting hoops in the back yard because his mom wanted him to get active at an early age. Little did she know that before middle school Wes would be one of the better players in a city known for producing basketball talent the way FedEx ships packages.

Wesley Williams plays for his school and travels the summer AAU circuit with the Memphis War Eagles 12 and under team, but even though his jump shot is already developed far beyond his years his parents approach his budding sports odyssey as just parents. Wes' parents make sure that he experiences healthy instruction in the neutral environment a gym provides, and not just the life X's and O's he digests at home. Not once has a referee had to give a seething glare in order to stop Wesley's mother Tracy from encouraging Wesley to rough house or take advantage of less-talented players.

Kelli Wheeler follows a similar approach with her two children. The author and freelance writer devotes a great deal of her time to enhancing the parental skills of the world through her website www.momservations.com, but she spends just as much time making sure that her children are actively enjoying sports in healthy, stress free environments around the Sacramento area.

The SacConnect blogger functions as the ultimate behind-the-scenes sports mom with sound advice, loads of encouragement, and creative energy. Wheeler's background as a track and field athlete also lends credence to her push for sports and activity at home. She is sure to encourage healthy eating and good sportsmanship for her soccer enthused son and daughter, but she is very mindful not to interfere with the coaching process to which her children are exposed.

"I always tell the kids, 'Healthy food and eating is fuel. You have to give your body what it needs if you're going to ask it to perform," said Wheeler during a 2011 interview. "When I'm tempted to offer constructive criticism I stop myself and first ask, 'Did you have fun out there?' I also always cheer, 'Get her done and have fun!'"

As a parent, you have to remember that ultimately it is your child's time to enjoy the gaming experience, and not yours to poke and prod them through. Provide encouragement and stay abreast of what is going on each time out, but make sure that you are not contradicting what your child's coach is trying to communicate when he or she is participating during practice and actual games.

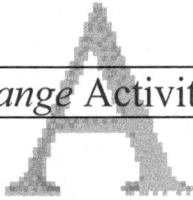

small change Activity to Kindle A Good Spirit:

Have your child write a "Thank You" note to himself/herself for anything in which he/she is grateful. It could be things such as; being a good friend, running an extra lap, sticking to his/her goals, or behaving well on a field trip. Be sure your child records it in his/her gratitude journal.

NOTES:

_____

_____

_____

_____

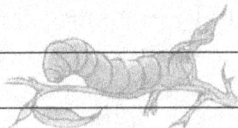
_____

_____

No Sports? No Problem!

Keep it simple, when you get too complex you forget the obvious.
~Al Maguire, NCAA Championship Basketball Coach

The body was made to move, and nobody has more fun teeter-tottering around than children. Once they learn to walk, they become little explorers, literally into everything they can get their hands and feet on.

Not every child will take a liking to sports, but there are still many ways to ensure physical activity and promote good health. Because your child has no interest in catching a fly ball doesn't mean that he or she has to miss out on physical activity fun.

Study after study indicates that today's youth may be the most inactive generation in history. Findings from a 2003 study conducted by the Henry J. Kaiser Family Foundation "Zero to Six: Media in the lives of Infants, Toddlers and Preschoolers," revealed that young children are spending as much media time including computers, TV and video games as playing outside. In the study, parents defended usage as an avenue to improve learning and stimulate intellectual development.

A five-year follow-up study revealed that with 24-hour media availability for children and teens, media entertainment among children and teens has risen dramatically. The January, 2010 report showed 8-18 year-olds devote an average of 7 hours and 38 minutes to using entertainment media on a typical day, which adds up to more than 53 hours weekly.

While technology is here to stay, and in many cases a positive tool in learning how to play certain sports, we remind parents that the body was not designed to be immobile. To return to the basics of encouraging children to play more and just have fun is a start in reversing the life-threatening trends of childhood obesity. Listed below are some of our tips, as well as suggestions from the National Association for Sport and Physical Education (NASPE) that will get your child headed in an active direction. By participating in these activities along with your child, you can kill three birds with one stone: The child is active; you are active; and you become his/her biggest role model when it comes to physical fitness.

Tips to Increase Physical Activity in Early Childhood

- Organize chase-and-flee games so that children increase their heart rates.
- If you don't live in a safe environment where children can play outside, take them to a park.
- Give children safe equipment and let them make up their own games.
- Buy them bikes, and tricycles and you ride or walk along with them (2 for 1).
- Play music and let children make up their own dance routines. You dance with them.
- Hold birthday parties outdoors and make physical activity the focus. (Scavenger hunts, hide-n-seek, the Blob, etc).

Excellent physical activity resources:
> www.headstartbodystart.org
> www.pecentral.org
> www.fitness.gov
> www.naeyc.org
> www/naspeinfo.org

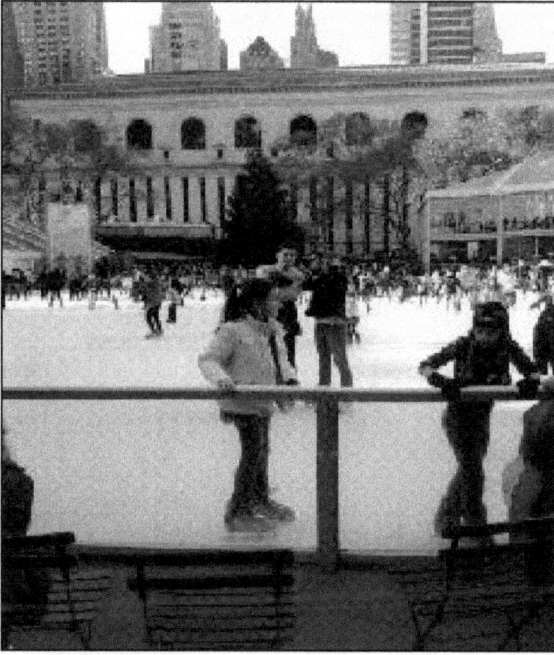

Ice skating is a fun, inexpensive
activity the entire family can enjoy!

small change Activity to Kindle A Good Spirit:

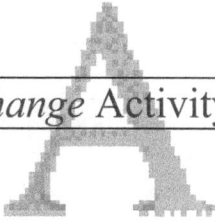

Have your child write one sports or personal fitness goal on a 3" x 5" index card and encourage her to look at it periodically while working to complete the goal. The goal could be as simple as "I will complete 10 pull-ups at the park playground," or "This season I am a Good Sport, win or lose."

Each time your child makes progress toward that goal have her list it in her gratitude journal. When your child completes the goal, have her file it away in a designated place and start on another. Goal setting promotes better focus, more organization, and increased self-esteem.

NOTES:

Tactical Closing

"Just Play. Have fun. Enjoy the Game."
~Michael Jordan, 6-Time NBA Champion

The closely linked trio of exercise, sports, and good health has been around for many centuries, but for such a long time in this country we have ignored the consequences of their absence in the lives of 21st Century youth in America. Despite having failed our young people in many ways pertaining to overall personal fitness, self-esteem and teamwork values, awareness has increased. With increased awareness also accompany expected changes.

More grocery carriers and fast food chains are cleaning up their acts, and professional sports leagues across the board have increased their respective involvements in righting the sports and fitness ship carrying too many immobile youngsters with worlds of physical potential. Now equipped with the small changes outlined for you in this book, the choice is yours as to which positive direction sports and physical activity steer your child.

Obstacles may arise as you and your child approach sports involvement and becoming more physically active, but the most important thing is to remember to keep plugging if it is truly a desire for you to have a healthy child interested in sports or just fun physical activity. Look at what you truly desire for your child and if it promotes good and causes no harm to you or your child, pursue it with your child in your highest and best consciousness. If you are unsure whether or not your desires for him/her are truly physically and mentally healthy, revisit Tactics One and Two.

Allow For Creativity

The places a child's mind takes him or her are limitless. If your child's personal sports bank also includes a vivid imagination, don't discourage it. Maybe your child thinks that having a bowl of his/her favorite cereal on the days of his/her meets makes her swim faster, or maybe he/she talks in third person as his/her favorite soccer star while taking shots on the side of the garage. Whatever his or her creative niche happens to be, promote the use of it. That imaginary genius that you see in his bedroom today could lead to a well-adjusted success story of tomorrow. Remember, even the greatest professional gamers imagined something while honing their respective sports crafts.

Stress Reverence

Sports reverence is simply holding your body, the game in which you play, and your opponent in high regard. Taking either component lightly could have negative repercussions including, not being physically ready to perform due to lack of sleep, forgetting the necessary equipment to participate, or displaying poor sportsmanship in the eyes of an opponent win or lose.

Remind your child often to always revere themselves, the activity of their choice, and the opposition, if one is present. He or she should refrain from trash-talking, intentionally harming an opponent, disrespecting authority figures, and slowing the body's development with harmful substances.

By stressing reverence for the body, the game, and the competition, your child will recognize the importance of all three meshing together cohesively so that he or she always accomplishes the ultimate goal when engaging in sports and physical activity…to have fun, enjoy it, and be fit.

NOTES:

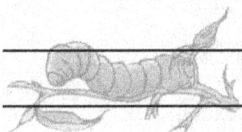

Bibliography

"Danica Patrick Poses for Got Milk," May 8, 2009,
http://www.autospies.com/news/Danica-Patrick- poses-for-Got-
Milk-43839/

Dugout Dispatch. "Q&A: Chadwick Boseman On Jackie Robinson
and 42," April 12, 2013,
http://www.sikids.com/blogs/2013/04/12/qa-chadwick-boseman-
on-jackie-robinson-and-42

Dyer, Wayne W. Ph.D. There's a Spiritual Solution to Every
Problem. New York. HarperCollins, 2001.

Goodman, Karon Phillips. Everyday Angels, Simple Ways to be an
Angel for Others Everyday. Uhrichsville, OH. Barbour, 2000.

"Lil Kickers Program Description." Accessed April 17, 2013,
http://www.lilkickers.com/program

"Physical Activity for Children: A Statement of Guidelines for
Children Ages 5 - 12, 2nd Edition." Accessed April 16, 2013,
http://www.aahperd.org/naspe/standards/nationalGuidelines/PA-
Children-5-12.cfm

"Promoting Physical Activity: A guide for Community Action."
US Department of Health and Human Services, Centers for Disease
Control, 1999. Human Kinetics. pg. xvii)

Russell, Cameron & Russell, Myrtle. small change, a 28 Day
Guide to Eating, Thinking, and Feeling Healthier. Jackson, TN.
Main Street, 2005.

Russell, Myrtle. Free Your Mind and the Best Will Follow.
Bloomington, IN. Balboa Press, 2012.

Simmons, Russell . Do You! 12 laws to Access the Power in You to Achieve Happiness and Success. New York. Penguin Group, 2007.

"What is Tee Ball," Accessed March 2, 2013, http://www.teeballusa.org/What_is_TBall.asp

Yaeger, Don. "Raising Champions." Success, October, 2010.

Photo Credits:

Photo 1(cover)-Mia Russell-Stocking
Photo 2: Microsoft ClipArt/used by permission
Photo 3-http://jasezone.com/wp-content/uploads/2013/04/youth-sports.jpg
Photo 3-Cameron T. Russell
Photo 4-Mia Russell-Stocking
Photo 5-Mia Russell-Stocking
Photo 6-Cameron T. Russell
Photo-7-Cameron T. Russell

About the Authors

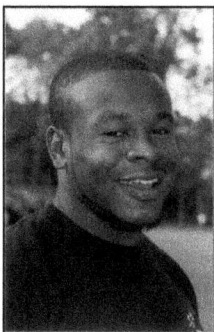

As a co-author of *small change* and University of Tennessee at Chattanooga graduate, Cameron has trained professionally in the fitness and sports arenas for thirteen years. He currently serves as a personal trainer/performance coach to professional athletes, as well as weekend warriors, expecting mothers, and youth looking to make lifestyle changes.

In addition to sports training and promoting health and wellness, Cameron serves on the Board of Directors for the North Side Neighborhood House in Chattanooga, edits sports for the *West Tennessee Examiner*, and has contributed fitness and sports articles to online publications www.livestrong.com and www.Examiner.com.

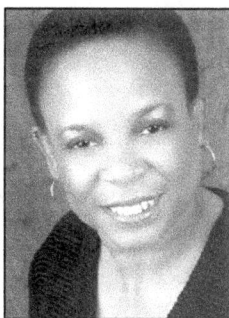

Myrtle Russell's career in health includes thirty years of service as nurse, educator, public health administrator, life coach, and writer. She currently serves as interim director for West TN Area Health Education Center, Inc., health editor for the *West Tennessee Examiner*, and spends the remainder of her time writing and coaching. She is the co-author of *small change: a 28-day guide to eating, thinking, and feeling healthier,* and has just released her second book, *Free Your Mind and the Best Will Follow*.